Natural Skin Care with Essential Oils

30 Best Anti-Aging Homemade Products

Table Of Contents

Introduction

We take the confusion out of natural beauty products...

By purchasing this book, you are embarking on a journey to holistic beauty and natural health to help you make your skin look healthy, young, and wrinkle-free.

We have taken our expertise and years of practice and knowledge gathering and put it in an easy-to-follow format. This means we explain the why and how an ingredient works. We all explain what to expect from the ingredients once you mix them into creams, facial masks and more.

Through essential oils and aromatherapy, you will learn how your skin changes as you age. You will also be introduced to how to change the recipes and products to suit your skin type and your age. As you age, so does your skin. We will help you make products to keep up with your skin changes and maintain its elasticity and health.

Attaining clear, healthy, younger looking skin doesn't have to be hard, confusing, or expensive. It can be fun and rewarding. It can also be educational as you will be learning about how to treat your skin from the inside out. This means some dietary changes.

Are you ready to learn about how to make beauty treatments at home? Let's get started.

Chapter 1 – Your Skin and You

Your skin, it's with you all your life. It goes through growth, the hormonal changes of puberty, and also protects you from infection and some illnesses. Your skin is the first line of defense your body has. Your body also shows the world what you have been through, your struggles, your stresses, and the environment you subject to every time you step out of the house.

When you're a child, you don't think about it much. You carry it with you everywhere you go and you subject it to winds as you ride your bike, run, or other activities. You don't worry about what you're doing to it, until you start puberty, and you look in the mirror. There it is, an oily spot on your face, your first pimple, or your notice your skin is dry, drier than you remember it.

As you get into in the work place and are subjected to supporting yourself, meeting deadlines, and dealing with the public at large, you experience stress. Your skin does as well. It begins to feel stretched, dry, and begins to develop wrinkles. You may even notice dark circles under your eyes. This is another phase of your life your face tells the world.

When you enter your fifties, your skin may begin to sage. It loses elasticity, the trait that allows your skin to bounce back and stay firm. The skin under your jaw sags. You begin to start looking your age. You wonder if there is a way to stop it, reverse it.

What you didn't realize...

Is that you can prevent it by keeping it moisturized, cleansed, and toned. You can do this by first making changes to your diet. Your skin health starts from within. The food you eat and the things you drink can affect your skin and how it ages.

Processed and fast food...

We all love convenience. We all love to grab something to eat and go on the way to work or running errands. You come home and a quick dinner is either out of a box or a frozen dinner. The problem with convenience is the chemicals which go into the foods you're putting into your body. Artificial additives can make your digestive system rebel, and when it rebels it can show on your face. Cold sores from indigestion, oilier skin and even break-outs can all be linked to the foods you eat.

Simply reading labels and cutting out these additives can be enough, as well as cutting out the greasy foods you're used to buying on a regular basis. Skipping the burger or fried chicken for salads, smoothies, and juices can help to keep your skin clear and healthy. It can even help to start reversing some of your skin problems.

Now, that you are working on the inside to take care of your skin, you're ready to learn about how to care for it on the outside, too.

Chapter 2 – Aromatherapy

When you first hear this word, you may be thinking diffusers, incense, and other things of that nature, but it is also massage lotions, massage oils, astringents, skin lotions and oils and a whole host of other things. It is also facial masks, moisturizers, cleansers, and baths.

Aromatherapy is the aspect of natural health which states that healing can come through the inhaling of aromas. These aromas are made by blending essential oils. Essential oils are the essence of the plant and often the most potent of preparations in the holistic field. Large amounts of a certain plant are either distilled or pressed for their pure oil, and it is this oil that is used in several remedies and applications.

The Applications

There are several ways one can use essential oils.

1. Diffuser, candle, or candle warmer.

This is the practice of placing the neat (undiluted oils) on a surface and then gently warming them to release their fragrance.

2. Bath/mineral salts

As the name states, you mix the oils with epsom salts, sea salts and a couple of other minerals to add to the bath for therapeutic effects.

3. Massage Oil/Lotion

This preparation is often used to loosen tight muscles, moisturize skin, and also deliver the healing effects of the essential oils.

4. Facial Masks

Used more commonly for spa treatments, a facial mask which has been infused with essential oils can heal rough, dry skin, treat acne, and help reduce fine lines and wrinkles. It is usually made by mixing clay, powdered herbs and other ingredients and then introducing the essential oils.

5. Astringents

These can be made with Witch Hazel, a natural cleanser. Depending on which essential oils are mixed into the Witch Hazel, you can not only cleanse skin, but you can also rebalance the pH of your skin to reduce oily patches and restore elasticity.

6. Soaps

Melt and pour soaps can be infused with essential oils for a healthier soap that can cleanse the entire body as well as your face. Melt and pour soaps contain more glycerin than the soaps you find in the store. Glycerin is the natural chemical in soap that provides moisture. Most commercially made soaps dry out the skin due to the fact most, if not all, of the glycerin has been processed out of the soap.

7. Facial Oils

I could have included this in the massage oil section, but facial oils are often used after you clean your face to help moisturize it. Depending on the carrier oil and essentials oils you blend together, they can make both night-time and day-time treatments for your skin.

Word to the wise

Not all essential oils agree with all skin types. A reputable vendor can help you find the essentials oil you need by helping you do a patch test to see if you have a reaction to the essential oil.

Do not, for any reason, use essential oils undiluted. There are a lot of websites which will tell you therapeutic grade essential oils can be used this way, but undiluted, or neat, essential oils can cause contact dermatitis and other skin reactions which can be unpleasant and may require a physician to treat. Always dilute your essential oils in carrier oils, or other mediums before using.

Chapter 3 – Essential and Carrier Oils

In this chapter, I will list the most common carrier and essential oils for home remedies and in making beauty products at home. If any of them have a risk of causing health issues to worsen, as in hypertension and the like, I will include that information as well. I include the Latin Name of the essential oil to help you purchase the correct one as there are many which can have similar names, but only one Latin designation.

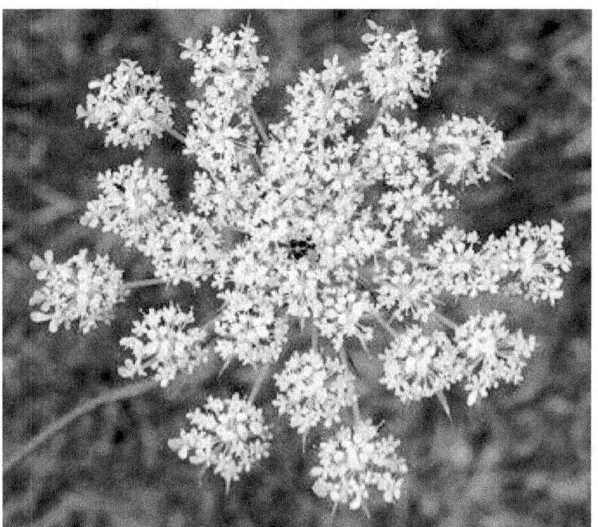

The essential oils

There are a certain set of essential oils used for beauty and skin care.

Carrot Seed Essential Oil

Daucus carota

When I say "carrot" you are probably thinking about the vegetable, and you would partially correct. It is Wild Carrot. It's also known as Queen Anne's Lace. This essential oil can be used to help in cases rashes, wrinkles, and returning the elasticity and healthy glow to mature skin types.

Frankincense

Boswellia carteri

Steeped in history and dated back to biblical times, this essential oil is more commonly used as an incense, but Frankincense is also added to blends and beauty products to help with blemishes, dry complexions, older skin, and the reduction of wrinkles.

Geranium

Pelargonium graveolens

Another on the list, geranium is used for many skin problems. It can help treat acne, broken capillaries, and also the problems that arise from mature skin. This means it helps to tone skin, minimize wrinkles, and reduces sagging.

Lavender Essential Oil

Lavendula angustifolia

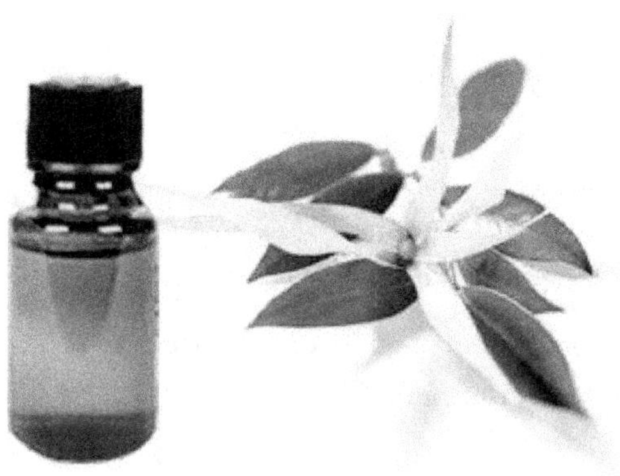

One of the more widely known essential oils, Lavender oil is versatile. It can blend with most other essential oils. It helps to treat acne, rosacea, age spots, and is good for maintaining all skin types by helping to balance the PH in the skin.

Myrrh

Commiphora myrrha

Another oil that has been around since biblical times, Myrrh is used in the aromatherapy world for chapped and dry skin, the maintenance of mature skin to keep its health and elasticity.

Neroli

Citrus aurantium var. amara

Otherwise known as Orange Blossom, this essential oil is touted for its ability to tone mature and sensitive skin. It can tone the complexion and reduce wrinkles.

Orange

Citrus sinesis

Sweet Orange is an essential oil is used to bring back the healthy glow in dull skin and balance an oily complexion.

Patchouli

Pogostemon cablin

Brought into popularity in the 1960's, this essential oil is added into blends to help shrink pores, helps to balance oily skin, and reduce wrinkles.

Rose

Rosa x damascena

The Damask Rose is prized for its properties regarding skin and the nervous system. It helps the repair broken capillaries, dry skin, and mature and sensitive complexions.

Sandalwood

Santalum album

This essential oil helps to treat chapped skin, greasy skin, and also helps to moisturize the skin.

Carrier Oils

Carrier oils are used in aromatherapy to help blend the oils and dilute them for use. There is a list of carrier oils that are used for beauty and skin care purposes.

Sweet Almond Oil

This is one of the more popular oils. It helps to relieve itching and dryness of the skin. This oil is good for all skin types.

Apricot Kernel Oil

This, like the oil above, is widely used in aromatherapy. It can be used in place of Sweet Almond oil if you are allergic to nuts. It is recommended if you have dry or sensitive skin.

Borage Oil

This oil is added to one of the two oils above for prematurely aged skin and also helps to stimulate healing of the skin. It is good for all skins types.

Carrot Oil

This oil is used for dry skin, prematurely aging skin, and helps to rejuvenate the skin. It is diluted with other carrier oils.

Evening Primrose Oil

Often used to balance hormone, Evening Primrose is also used to prevent prematurely aging skin. It is often diluted with other carrier oils.

Wheatgerm Oil

This oil helps to tone prematurely aged skin and is good for all skin types. It is also diluted in a blend.

Other things you can use.

There are other ingredients you can use to dilute essential oils.

Base lotion

You can find unscented, plain lotion online to make your own lotions. This is a good way to make moisturizers for your face and body.

Witch Hazel

This is touched in a previous chapter. You can dilute essential oils in Witch Hazel to use as an astringent and other skin tonics.

Bentonite Clay

This mineral clay is used as a base for facial masks. It helps to detoxify the skin.

French Clay

This is used like bentonite clay.

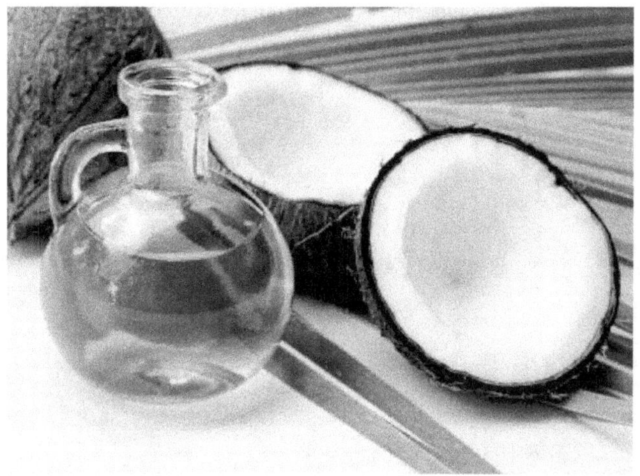

Base liquid soap

You can find plain liquid soap online to make a facial cleanser tailored to your skin complexion.

Tips on making your own blends.

In another chapter, we will include recipes, but if you are interested in making your own blends and products, here are a few tips.

Add six drops of essential oil per one tablespoon of carrier oil or carrier oil blend. This also works if you are adding essential oils to lotions and soaps.

Heavier essential oils are added in smaller amounts than lighter ones. Heavier essential oils include essential oils from herbs and tree saps. Heavier oils are also essential oils from bark.

Lighter essential oils are oils from fruit rinds, leaves, and flower petals.

Carrier oils other than Sweet Almond or Apricot oil should be added in ratios of 10 percent.

It is best to store essential oil blends in glass bottles and jars with dark colors. The more light you expose the essential oils to, the faster they lose their effectiveness. Keep them in a cool dark place.

Chapter 4 – Essential oils and your age

As we age, so does your skin. Your skin's needs change as you age in order to keep it healthy, glowing, and firm. This chapter will help you break down which essential oils are more effective for your age.

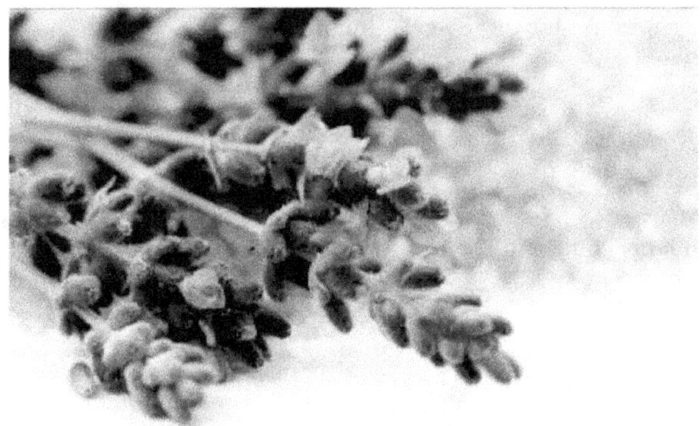

Twenties

You can maintain your youthful appearance at this age by using the following essential oils:

Carrot Seed

Geranium

Lavender

Neroli

You can use Sweet Almond, or apricot oil with Evening Primrose oil.

Thirties

Your body is hitting its peak. Your skin is starting show some signs of age, but you can use the following oils to turn back time:

Patchouli

Rose

Carrot Seed

Palma Rosa (an oil that is used to reduce wrinkles and soften skin)

You can use Borage seed oil to your Sweet Almond or Apricot Kernel.

Forties

You're more mature and so is your skin. You may notice wrinkles at this age and some dryness. You may also start to see some sagging.

Carrot Seed

Frankincense

Lavender

Neroli

You can use Borage seed, Carrot Oil, Evening Primrose, or Wheatgerm oil to your lighter carrier oils.

Fifties

There are a few more wrinkles and it may be sagging a little more and you're also noticing age spots and other symptoms due to aging.

Carrot Seed

Lavender

Myrrh

Neroli

Rose

Evening Primrose and Borage Seed oils are especially good for this age range.

Chapter 5 – Facial Cleansers

It's been a long day, you're ready for bed. You've taken your shower and now you're going to cleanse your skin before resting your head for the night.

Soaps

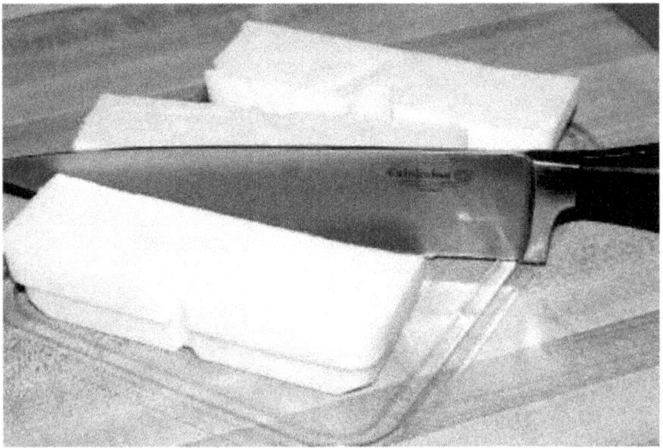

Your face is more sensitive than the rest of your body, and it deserves special treatment. The soaps you use on your body can take its toll on your face.

Oily Skin Melt and Pour soap

4 ounces of Goat's Milk Melt and Pour soap

2 tablespoons of used coffee grinds.

2 tablespoons of ground oats

25 Drops of Orange essential oil

25 Drops of Lavender Essential oil

20 Drops of Geranium essential oil

20 Drops of Patchouli essential oil

10 Drops of Frankincense essential oil

- In a double boiler melt the soap

- Add the coffee and ground oats

- Pour the soap into the molds.

- Mix the essential oils together

- Add the essential oils when the soap is warm but still viable

The coffee grinds will act as an astringent and an exfoliants. The oats will help to absorb excess oil.

Melt and Pour Soap for Dry Skin

4 Ounces of Olive Oil

2 tablespoons of Kelp (natural silicon and minerals that are good for the skin)

25 Drops of Lavender essential oil

25 Drops of Geranium essential oil

20 Drops of Rose essential oil

20 Drops of Myrrh essential oil

10 Drops of Frankincense essential oil

- Melt the soap in a double boiler

- Add the Kelp

- Pour the soap into molds.

- Mix all the essential oils

- Equally add the essentials oils to the soap when it is warm and still viable.

Skin Balancing Melt and Pour Soap

2 Ounce of Goat's Milk Melt and Pour

2 Ounces of Olive Oil Melt and Pour

2 Tablespoons of Coffee Grinds

1 Tablespoons of Kelp

25 Drops of Orange essential oil

25 Drops of Geranium essential oil

20 Drops of Patchouli essential oil

20 Drops of Rose essential oil

10 Drops of Myrrh essential oil

- Melt the soap in a double boiler

- Add the grinds and kelp

- Pour the soap into molds

- Mix the essential oils

- Add the essential oils when the soap is warm but still viable.

Liquid soaps

You can use liquid soaps on your skin to cleanse and balance your skin. You can purchase plain liquid base for you soap recipes online.

Soothing Skin Soap

4 Ounces of Liquid soap base

25 Drops Lavender essential oil

20 Drops Geranium essential oil

15 Drops Patchouli essential oil

15 Drops Orange essential oil

15 Drops Neroli essential oil

10 Drops Myrrh essential oil

Detox Soap

4 Ounces of Liquid soap Base

30 Drops Peppermint essential oil

25 Drops Lavender essential oil

30 Drops Rose essential oil

15 Drops of Sandalwood

Dry Skin Soap

4 Ounces of Liquid Soap Base

30 Drops of Lavender essential oil

25 Drops of Rose essential oil

25 Drops of Neroli essential oil

20 Drops of Myrrh essential oil

Oily Skin Soap

4 Ounces Liquid Soap Base

25 Drops Orange essential oil

25 Drops Carrot Seed essential oil

25 Drops of Sandalwood essential oil

25 Drops Geranium

Invigorating Soap

4 Ounces Liquid Base Soap

30 Drops Peppermint essential oil

30 Drops Orange essential oil

20 Drops Neroli essential oil

20 Drops Sandalwood essential oil

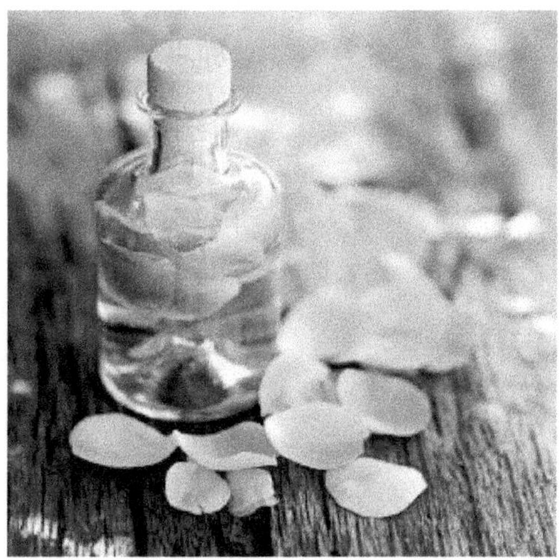

Astringents

This is the natural next step in the cleansing process. It can remove the dirt and oils the soap may have missed. Once you've mixed the astringent, you can add it to a bottle you've previously emptied. Use a cotton ball to apply the astringent.

The base for the astringent is one ounce of Apple Cider Vinegar and three ounces of Witch Hazel. Make sure you add the essential oils to the Apple Cider Vinegar before you add the Witch Hazel. The Cider Vinegar will help emolliate the essential oils so they can mix more effectively with the Witch Hazel.

Twenties

3 Ounces of Witch Hazel

1 Ounce Apple Cider Vinegar

20 Drops Peppermint essential oil (antiseptic properties)

20 Drops Lavender essential oil

20 Drops Carrot Seed oil

20 Drops Geranium

- Mix the essential oils into the vinegar

- Add the infused vinegar to the Witch Hazel

- Place in a dark colored bottle.

- Apply a small of the astringent to a cotton ball and cleanse face as normal.

Thirties

2 Ounces of Witch Hazel

1 Ounce Rose Water (Soothes and tones skin)

1 Ounce Apple Cider Vinegar

20 Drops Palma Rosa essential oil

20 Drops Rose essential oil

10 Drops Patchouli essential oil

10 Drops Sandalwood essential oil

20 Drops Peppermint essential oil

- Mix the Essential oils in the vinegar

- Mix the Rose water and Witch Hazel

- Mix all the ingredients together.

- Place them in a dark colored bottle.

- Place a few drops on a cotton ball as you would any other astringent.

Forties

2 Ounces Rose Water

1 Ounce Witch Hazel

1 Ounce Apple Cider Vinegar

20 Drops Neroli essential oil

20 Drops Lavender essential oil

10 Drops Patchouli essential oil

10 Drops Frankincense essential oil

20 Drops of Carrot essential oil

- Mix the essential oils in the vinegar

- Add the Witch Hazel and Rose Water

- Pour into a dark colored bottle.

- Put a few drops on a cotton ball and apply as normal.

Fifties

2 Ounces of Rose Water

1 Ounce of Witch Hazel

1 Ounce of Apple Cider Vinegar

20 Drops Lavender essential oil

20 Drops Neroli essential oil

10 Drops Sandalwood essential oil

10 Drops Geranium essential oil

10 Drops Myrrh essential oil

10 Drops Rose essential oil

- Mix the essential oils and the vinegar
- Add the rest of the ingredients
- Pour into a dark colored bottle
- Use as you normally would

Chapter 6 – Moisturizers

After you have washed, and applied the astringent, you may feel your skin is a little dry. This is why the next step in your regimen should be to moisturize your skin. This is especially true if you have oily skin as well as dry.

When your skin is freshly cleaned, it is dry because you have cleansed the dirt and with it, your natural oils that help to keep your skin smooth and healthy.

If you have oily skin, may have noticed your skin gets oily relatively quickly after it has been cleaned. This is because your skin is trying to pull moisture back into your skin.

There are two ways to add moisture back into your skin:

- Making your lotion

- Making a massage oil

This is very important as some oils can be lighter than lotions for your face. These would be perfect for oily skin types.

Facial moisturizing oils

Twenties

3 1/2 Ounces Sweet Almond or Apricot Kernel Oil

1/2 Ounce Evening Primrose Oil

20 Drops Lavender essential oil

20 Drops Geranium essential oil

10 Drops Neroli essential oil

10 Drops Carrot Seed oil

10 Drops Orange essential oil

10 Drops Sandalwood essential oil

- Mix all the ingredients together

- Pour into a dark colored bottle

- Apply using a cotton ball

Thirties

3 1/2 Ounces of Sweet Almond or Apricot Kernel oil

1/2 Ounce of Borage Seed oil

20 Drops Palma Rosa essential oil

20 Drops of Rose essential oil

10 Drops Carrot Seed essential oil

10 Drops Patchouli essential oil

10 Drops Myrrh essential oil

10 Drops Lavender essential oil

- Follow the above instructions.

Forties

2 Tablespoons of Carrot oil

2 Tablespoons Borage Seed oil

Sweet Almond or Apricot Kernel oil

20 Drops Lavender essential oil

20 Drops Neroli essential oil

10 Drops Carrot Seed essential oil

10 Drops Frankincense essential oil

10 Drops Geranium essential oil

10 Drops Orange essential oil

- Follow the above instructions

Fifties

2 Tablespoons Evening Primrose oil

2 Tablespoons Wheatgerm oil

2 Tablespoons Borage Seed oil

Sweet Almond or Apricot Kernel oil

20 Drops Lavender essential oil

20 Drops Rose essential oil

10 Drops Neroli essential oil

10 Drops Myrrh essential oil

10 Drops Sandalwood essential oil

10 Drops Geranium essential oil

To make the lotions, just mix the essential oils first and then add them to four ounces of unscented plain base lotion.

Chapter 7 - Facial Masks

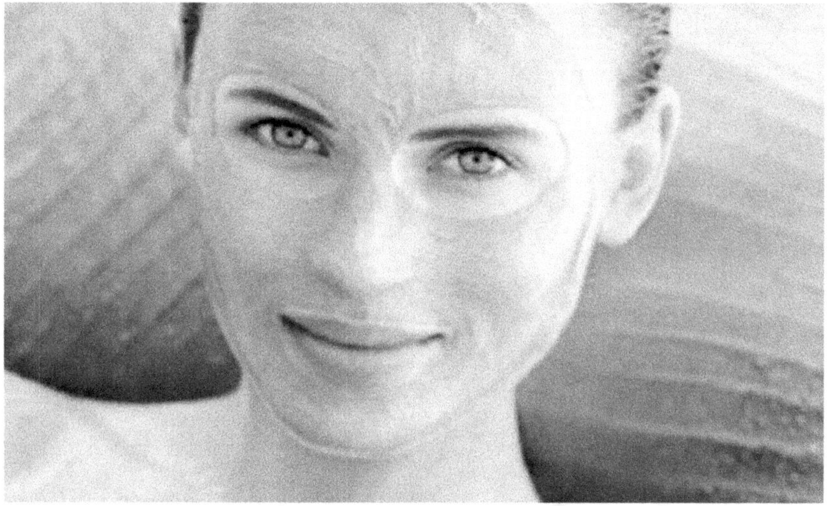

Facial masks are used to detoxify the skin as well as tone the skin, and promote the healing of skin ravaged by the environment and stress.

To use the masks, simply moisten three tablespoons of the mask with warm water and then knead in 6-10 drops of the essential oil blend. Spread it evenly on your skin and allow it to dry. This should take about ten minutes. You then remoisten it to either rinse it off, or you can use it as a scrub before you rinse it off. Always follow-up mask use with an astringent and then a moisturizer.

Below, I am listing the different types of masks you can use. You can add the above essential oil blends from the previous chapter to the masks before applying it.

Detoxifying Mask

1/4 Cup Bentonite Clay Powder

1/8 Cup Lavender flowers

1/8 Cup Ground Oats

1/8 Cup Spirulina

Skin Balancing Mask

1/8 Cup Bentonite Clay Powder

1/8 Cup French Clay Powder

1/8 Cup Peppermint leaves

1/8 Cup Lavender Flowers

1/8 Cup Dried Orange Zest

Oily Skin Mask

1/4 Cup Ground Oats

1/8 Cup Bentonite Clay Powder

1/8 Cup Dried Lemon Zest

1/8 Cup Kelp Powder

Dry Skin Mask

1/4 Cup Bentonite Clay Powder

1/8 Cup Kelp Powder

1/8 Cup Lavender Flowers

1/8 Cup Geranium Flowers, ground

Here are some blends that you can mix and max with the masks above.

Detox Blend

1 teaspoon Borage seed oil

1 tbsp coconut oil, melted

4 Drops Peppermint essential oil

2 Drops Orange essential oil

2 Drops Lavender essential oil

Dry Skin Blend

1/4 tsp Carrot Oil

2 Tablespoons Sweet Almond or Apricot Kernel oil

6 Drops Lavender essential oil

4 Drops Myrrh essential oil

2 Drops Rose essential oil

Oily Skin Blend

2 Tablespoons of Sweet Almond Oil

4 Drops Orange essential oil

4 Drops Lavender essential oil

2 Drops Patchouli essential oil

2 Drops Sandalwood essential oil

Chapter 8 - Mineral Baths

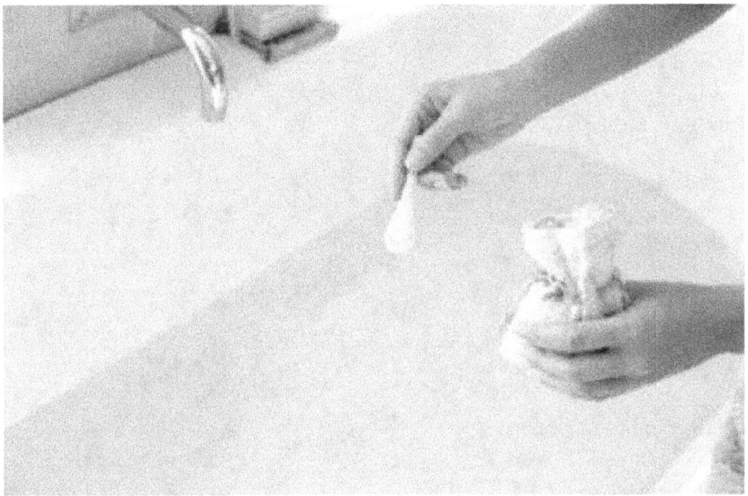

The best way to take of your body at the end of day is to soak in a mineral salt bath. You can also take an oatmeal bath if you have hypertension or dry skin.

To make the baths:

- Mix all the dry ingredients first

- Mix all the liquid ingredients.

- Slowly add the liquid ingredients into the dry

- Mix well and place in a container with a tight lid overnight.

Here is your basic recipe for the baths:

Mineral Bath

1 Cup Epsom Salt

1/2 Cup Magnesium flakes

1/2 Cup Pink Sea Salt

1/4 Cup Borax

1/4 Cup Baking Soda

Oatmeal Bath

1 Cup Ground Steel Cut Oats

1/2 Cup Borax

1/4 Cup Baking Soda

Detox Bath

1/2 Cup Powdered Echinacea

3 Tbsp Coconut oil

3 tbsp Sweet Almond or Apricot Kernel oil

12 Drops Lavender essential oil

6 Drops Peppermint essential oil

4 Drops Orange essential oil

2 Drops Sandalwood essential oil

Dry Skin Bath

1/2 Cup Lavender Flowers

3 Tbsp Sweet Almond oil

3 Tbsp Evening Primrose oil

12 Drops of Geranium essential oil

6 Drops of Patchouli essential oil

4 Drops of Myrrh essential oil

2 Drops Frankincense essential oil

Oily Skin Bath

3 Tbsp Wheatgerm oil

3 Tbsp Sweet Almond oil

12 Drops Orange essential oil

6 Drops Peppermint essential oil

6 Drops Sandalwood essential oil

Relaxing Bath

6 Tbsp Sweet Almond Oil or Apricot Kernel oil

12 Drops of Lavender essential oil

12 Drops of Geranium essential oil

Energizing Bath

6 Tbsp Sweet Almond or Apricot Kernel oil

12 Drops Orange essential oil

12 Drops Peppermint oil

Conclusion

There are a myriad of ways you can use essential oils. Try some of your own blends and mixes. If you want more information, there are online forums and groups you can join to get more information and advice on aromatherapy and essential oils.

I hope this book provided you with enough information to get you started on your way to making your own beauty products.

FREE Bonus Reminder

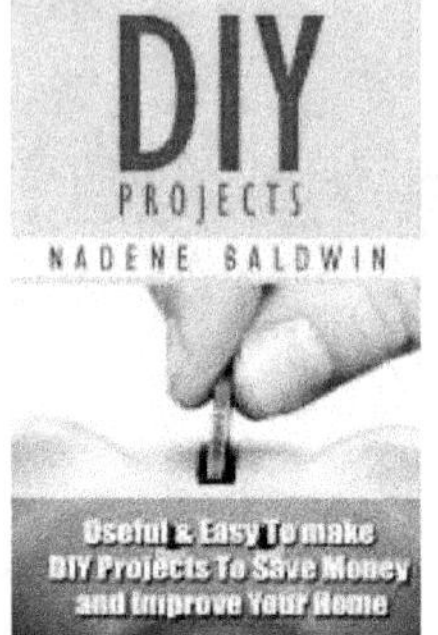

If you have not grabbed it yet, please go ahead and download your special bonus report *"DIY Projects. 13 Useful & Easy To Make DIY Projects To Save Money & Improve Your Home!"*
Simply Click the Button Below

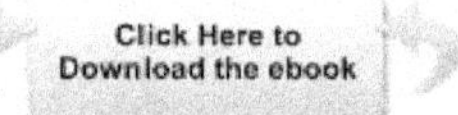

OR **Go to This Page**
http://diyhomecraft.com/free

BONUS #2: More Free & Discounted Books or Products
Do you want to receive more Free/Discounted Books or Products?
We have a mailing list where we send out our new Books or Products when they go free or with a discount on Amazon. Click on the link below to sign up for Free & Discount Book & Product Promotions.
=> Sign Up for Free & Discount Book & Product Promotions <=

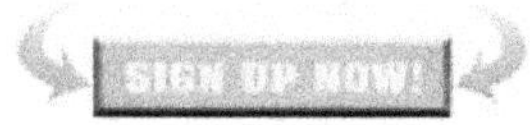

OR Go to this URL
http://zbit.ly/1WBb1Ek

www.ingramcontent.com/pod-product-compliance
Lightning Source LLC
Chambersburg PA
CBHW060817260726
48660CB00002B/1000

ISBN 9781979301978

9 781979 301978

Homemade Laundry Detergent

30 Recipes of Safe DIY Detergent

Carla Williams

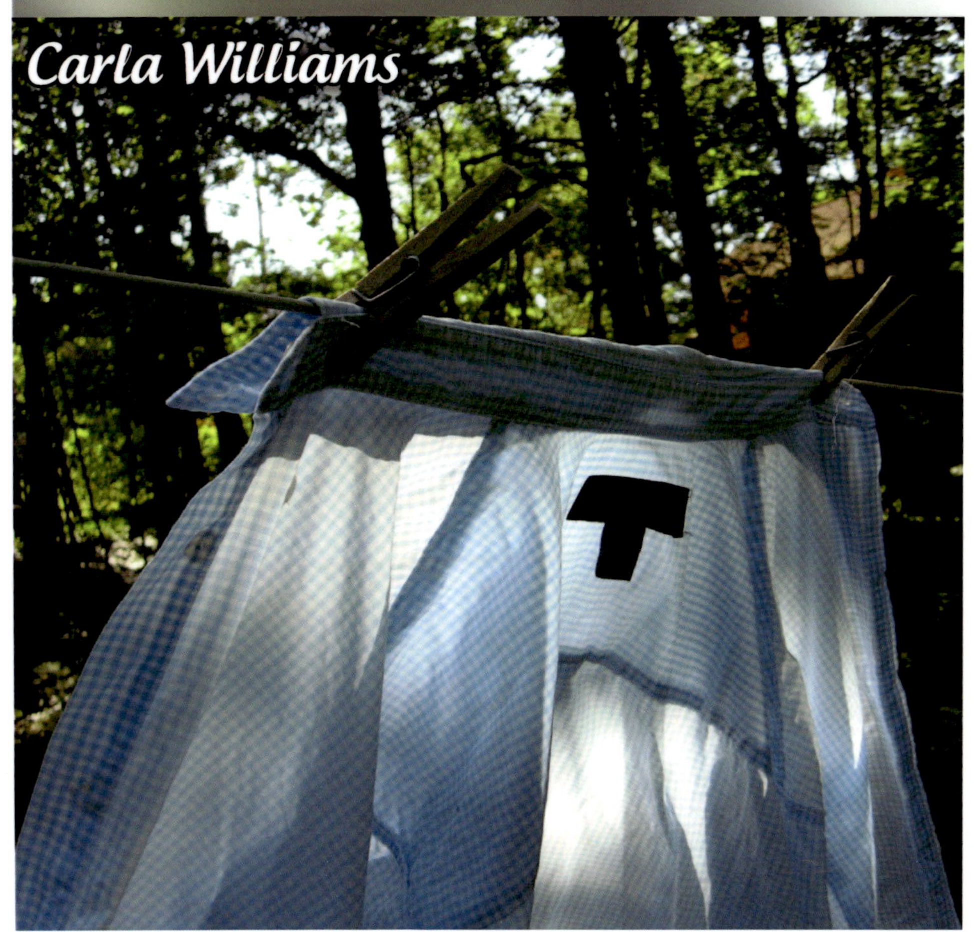